Anti Inflammatory Diet Guide For Beginners

A Beginners Guide To Anti-Inflammatory Diet Plus Simplified Meal Plans And Easy Recipes To Nourish The Immune System

Ryan Weimann Bailey

Table of Contents

Introduction

Inflammation is a natural process that the body uses to protect itself from harmful stimuli, such as pathogens, damaged cells, or irritants. It involves a complex series of chemical and cellular responses that can help to isolate and eliminate the source of the problem. Inflammation is a normal and essential part of the body's immune response, but when it becomes chronic or excessive, it can lead to tissue damage and a range of health problems.

The anti-inflammatory diet is not a specific, rigid diet plan. Instead, it is a dietary pattern that emphasizes whole, nutrient-dense foods while limiting or avoiding processed and inflammatory foods. The diet is high in fruits and vegetables, whole grains, healthy fats, and lean proteins, while being low in added sugars, trans fats, and saturated fats.

The anti-inflammatory diet is based on the idea that chronic inflammation in the body is linked to many health problems, including heart disease, diabetes, cancer, and autoimmune disorders. By following an anti-inflammatory diet, individuals can reduce inflammation in the body, which may help prevent or manage these conditions.

Some common foods that are recommended on an anti-inflammatory diet include leafy greens, berries, nuts and seeds, fatty fish, olive oil, and herbs and spices like turmeric, ginger, and garlic. Foods that should be avoided or limited include processed and packaged foods, high-sugar foods and drinks, trans fats and saturated fats, dairy products, and red and processed meat.

Research on the anti-inflammatory diet is ongoing, but some studies have shown that it may be effective for reducing inflammation and improving various health outcomes. However, it's important to note that the anti-inflammatory diet should not be used as a substitute for medical treatment or advice. Always consult with a healthcare professional or registered dietitian before making significant changes to your diet or lifestyle.

CHAPTER ONE

How can inflammation affect your health?

Chronic inflammation has been linked to a variety of health conditions, including cardiovascular disease, type 2 diabetes, cancer, arthritis, and Alzheimer's disease, among others. Inflammation can damage tissues and organs over time, leading to pain, swelling, and decreased function. It can also disrupt the body's hormonal and metabolic processes, contributing to weight gain, insulin resistance, and other health problems.

An anti-inflammatory diet is a way of eating that emphasizes whole, nutrient-dense foods that can help to reduce inflammation in the body. It typically includes a variety of fruits and vegetables, whole grains, lean protein sources, healthy fats, and anti-inflammatory herbs and spices. The goal of an anti-inflammatory diet is to reduce the consumption of pro-inflammatory foods, such as refined sugars, saturated and trans fats, and processed foods, while increasing the intake of foods that can help to reduce inflammation, such as omega-3 fatty acids, fiber, and antioxidants.

Foods to include in an anti-inflammatory diet

Fruits and vegetables

Fruits and vegetables are an important part of an anti-inflammatory diet because they are high in fiber, antioxidants, and other nutrients that can help to reduce inflammation. Berries, leafy greens, broccoli, and tomatoes are particularly good choices because they are high in antioxidants and phytochemicals that have been shown to have anti-inflammatory effects.

Whole grains

Whole grains are another important component of an anti-inflammatory diet because they are high in fiber and other nutrients that can help to reduce inflammation. Whole grain options include brown rice, quinoa, barley, and whole wheat bread. Avoid refined grains such as white bread and pasta, which can contribute to inflammation.

Healthy fats

Healthy fats, such as those found in fish, nuts, seeds, and avocados, are an important part of an anti-inflammatory diet. Omega-3 fatty acids, in particular, have been shown to have anti-inflammatory effects. Good sources of omega-3s include fatty fish (such as salmon and sardines), chia seeds, and flaxseeds.

Lean protein

Lean protein sources such as chicken, turkey, fish, legumes, and tofu can help to reduce inflammation and promote healthy muscles and tissues. Choose lean options and avoid processed meats, which can contribute to inflammation.

Spices and herbs

Many spices and herbs have anti-inflammatory properties and can add flavor and variety to an anti-inflammatory diet. Turmeric, ginger, garlic, cinnamon, and rosemary are just a few examples of spices and herbs that have been shown to have anti-inflammatory effects. Use them to season dishes instead of relying on salt or high-fat condiments.

Foods to avoid in an anti-inflammatory diet

Processed and packaged foods

Processed and packaged foods often contain high levels of sugar, salt, and unhealthy fats, and can contribute to inflammation in the body. These foods may also contain artificial additives and preservatives that can be harmful to health. Examples of processed and packaged foods to avoid include chips, crackers, cookies, and pre-packaged meals.

High-sugar foods and drinks

High-sugar foods and drinks, such as soda, candy, and baked goods, can cause inflammation in the body and contribute to a range of health problems, including obesity and type 2 diabetes. Limit your intake of these foods and drinks as much as possible, and opt for whole fruits instead of fruit juices.

Trans fats and saturated fats

Trans fats and saturated fats are unhealthy fats that can contribute to inflammation in the body. Trans fats are often found in processed foods, fried foods, and baked goods, while saturated fats are found in animal products such as meat and dairy. Limit your intake of these fats as much as possible, and opt for healthier fats such as olive oil, avocado, and nuts.

Dairy products

Dairy products can be pro-inflammatory for some people, especially those who are lactose intolerant or have a dairy allergy. Additionally, some studies suggest that milk proteins may trigger an immune response in some people, leading to inflammation. Consider alternatives such as nut milks or lactose-free dairy products if you experience digestive issues or other symptoms after consuming dairy.

Red and processed meat

Red and processed meats, such as beef, pork, and sausage, are high in saturated fat and can contribute to inflammation in the body. These meats have also been linked to an increased risk of heart disease, cancer, and other health problems. Choose lean protein sources such as chicken, fish, or legumes instead.

CHAPTER TWO

Tips for following an anti-inflammation

Some tips for following an anti-inflammation are:

Plan ahead

Planning your meals and snacks in advance can help you stay on track with an anti-inflammatory diet. Set aside time each week to plan out your meals, make a shopping list, and prep ingredients ahead of time. This can help you avoid unhealthy options and make it easier to stick to your dietary goals.

Read food labels

Read food labels Reading food labels can help you identify foods that are high in unhealthy fats, added sugars, and artificial additives. Look for products that are low in saturated and trans fats, contain no added sugars, and are free from artificial preservatives or colors.

Cook at home

Cooking at home allows you to control the ingredients and preparation methods used in your meals. It also allows you to experiment with new recipes and flavors, and can be a fun way to explore new foods. Try preparing simple meals that feature lean protein, whole grains, and plenty of fruits and vegetables.

Experiment with new recipes and flavors

One of the keys to following an anti-inflammatory diet is variety. Experimenting with new recipes and flavors can help you discover new favorite foods and keep your meals interesting. Look for recipes that feature anti-inflammatory ingredients such as leafy greens, berries, and fatty fish, and try incorporating new spices and herbs into your meals for added flavor and health benefits.

Sample meal plan for an anti-inflammatory diet

Breakfast

- Overnight oats made with rolled oats, almond milk, chia seeds, and topped with fresh berries and sliced almonds
- Green smoothie made with spinach, kale, banana, and almond butter

Lunch

- Grilled chicken breast with roasted sweet potatoes and steamed broccoli

- Quinoa salad with chopped vegetables, avocado, and a citrus vinaigrette dressing

Dinner

- Baked salmon with roasted Brussels sprouts and wild rice
- Lentil soup with a side salad of mixed greens and vegetables
- Snacks
- Apple slices with almond butter
- Carrot sticks with hummus
- Greek yogurt with fresh berries and nuts

Supplements for an anti-inflammatory diet

Some supplements that may support an anti-inflammatory diet:

Omega-3 fatty acids

Omega-3 fatty acids are a type of healthy fat that can help reduce inflammation in the body. You can get omega-3s from fatty fish such as salmon and mackerel, as well as from supplements like fish oil or krill oil.

Probiotics

Probiotics are beneficial bacteria that live in your gut and can help improve digestion and reduce inflammation. You can get probiotics from fermented foods like yogurt, kefir, and sauerkraut, as well as from supplements.

Turmeric and curcumin

Turmeric is a spice that contains a powerful anti-inflammatory compound called curcumin. You can add turmeric to your food or take curcumin supplements to help reduce inflammation in the body.

Ginger

Ginger is another spice that has anti-inflammatory properties. It may help reduce inflammation in the body and alleviate symptoms of digestive disorders such as nausea and bloating. You can add ginger to your food or take ginger supplements.

Vitamin D

Vitamin D is an important nutrient that plays a role in immune function and reducing inflammation. You can get vitamin D from sunlight, certain foods like fatty fish and fortified dairy products, and supplements.

It's important to note that while supplements can be helpful in supporting an anti-inflammatory diet, they should not be used as a substitute for a healthy, balanced diet. Consult with a healthcare professional or registered dietitian before taking any supplements to ensure they are safe and appropriate for you.

CHAPTER THREE

Advantages of an anti-inflammatory diet

Reduced inflammation: One of the main benefits of an anti-inflammatory diet is that it can help to reduce inflammation in the body. Chronic inflammation is linked to a variety of health problems, so reducing inflammation can improve overall health.

Improved heart health: An anti-inflammatory diet can also improve heart health by reducing risk factors for heart disease such as high blood pressure and high cholesterol.

Better digestion: An anti-inflammatory diet can improve digestion by promoting the growth of beneficial gut bacteria and reducing inflammation in the gut.

Weight loss: Following an anti-inflammatory diet can lead to weight loss, as many of the recommended foods are low in calories and high in nutrients.

Reduced risk of chronic diseases: An anti-inflammatory diet can reduce the risk of chronic diseases such as cancer, diabetes, and Alzheimer's disease.

Disadvantages of an anti-inflammatory diet

Restrictive: An anti-inflammatory diet can be restrictive, as it limits certain foods such as processed and packaged foods, high-sugar foods and drinks, and dairy products.

Requires planning and preparation: Anti-inflammatory diet requires planning and preparation as many convenience foods are not allowed.

Cost: Some of the recommended foods on an anti-inflammatory diet, such as organic fruits and vegetables, can be expensive.

Diseases that can benefit from an anti-inflammatory diet

Arthritis: An anti-inflammatory diet can help to reduce inflammation in the joints and improve symptoms of arthritis.

Asthma: An anti-inflammatory diet can reduce inflammation in the airways and improve symptoms of asthma.

Inflammatory bowel disease (IBD): An anti-inflammatory diet can reduce inflammation in the gut and improve symptoms of IBD.

Diabetes: An anti-inflammatory diet can improve blood sugar control and reduce the risk of complications in people with diabetes.

Heart disease: An anti-inflammatory diet can reduce risk factors for heart disease such as high blood pressure and high cholesterol, and improve overall heart health.

Control of anti-inflammatory dietdiseases

An anti-inflammatory diet can help in controlling various chronic diseases. Chronic inflammation has been linked to several chronic conditions such as heart disease, diabetes, arthritis, and even cancer. By following an anti-inflammatory diet, you can lower inflammation levels in your body, which can help manage and reduce the symptoms of these chronic diseases.

Heart disease is a leading cause of death worldwide, and chronic inflammation is a significant risk factor for the development of heart disease. By reducing inflammation levels, an anti-inflammatory diet can help lower the risk of heart disease. Studies have shown that following an anti-inflammatory diet, such as the Mediterranean diet, can help reduce the risk of heart disease by lowering cholesterol and blood pressure levels.

Inflammation is also linked to diabetes, and an anti-inflammatory diet can help manage blood sugar levels and insulin sensitivity. Foods that are high in refined carbohydrates and sugar can cause inflammation in the body, leading to insulin resistance and type 2 diabetes. An anti-inflammatory diet, on the other hand, emphasizes whole foods, including fruits, vegetables, whole grains, and lean protein, which can help manage blood sugar levels.

Arthritis is a condition characterized by joint inflammation, pain, and stiffness. An anti-inflammatory diet can help reduce inflammation and pain associated with arthritis. Foods that are high in sugar, refined carbohydrates, and saturated fats can cause inflammation, leading to joint pain and swelling. An anti-inflammatory diet can help reduce inflammation levels and improve joint health by including foods such as fatty fish, nuts, and berries.

In addition to these chronic diseases, an anti-inflammatory diet can also help reduce the risk of cancer. Chronic inflammation has been linked to the development of cancer, and an anti-inflammatory diet can help lower inflammation levels in the body, reducing the risk of cancer. By including foods rich in antioxidants, such as fruits and vegetables, an anti-inflammatory diet can also help protect against cancer by reducing oxidative stress in the body.

However, it is important to note that an anti-inflammatory diet may not be suitable for everyone. People with certain medical conditions, such as kidney disease, may need to limit their intake of certain foods, such as those high in potassium or phosphorus. Additionally, an anti-inflammatory diet may not be appropriate for people with eating disorders or a history of disordered eating. It is always important to consult a healthcare professional before making significant dietary changes.

Conclusion

Anti-inflammatory diet emphasizes whole, nutrient-dense foods while avoiding processed and inflammatory foods. By following this dietary pattern, individuals may experience reduced inflammation, improved heart health, better digestion, weight loss, and a reduced risk of chronic diseases.

Transitioning to an anti-inflammatory diet can be challenging, but starting slow and making gradual changes can make the transition more manageable. It's important to plan ahead, read food labels, cook at home, and experiment with new recipes and flavors.

Additionally, incorporating supplements such as omega-3 fatty acids, probiotics, turmeric, ginger, and vitamin D may further enhance the anti-inflammatory benefits of the diet.

THE END